I0440124

Facelift by Acupressure

Beauty and Vitality at Your Fingertips

by Ina C. Niemann

Copyright 2014 Ina C. Niemann

All Rights Reserved

Disclaimer

The author does not dispense medical advice or prescribe the use of any technique as a form of treatment for physical or emotional issues without the advice of a physician, either directly or indirectly.

This book is not intended to replace the services of a licensed healthcare professional in the diagnosis or treatment of illness. Any application of the material set forth in the following pages is at the reader's discretion and sole responsibility.

Dedication

To my husband and kids for their love, support and guidance.

Table of Content

Introduction

Even though the skin is our largest organ – about 2 square meter – the part on our face accounts for four and a half percent only. Yet it attracts more attention, generates more concern and feeds more commercial enterprises than any other part of the body. We obviously find it difficult to accept the marks of time gracefully because they affect the way we present ourselves to the world.

Throughout the ages, women have been preoccupied with the attempt to halt or at least slow down the signs of ageing – with limited success only. Furthermore, our perception of age is changing continuously. Instead of being associated with seniority, experience and wisdom, old age has become something to be shunned and no effort is spared to keep our face looking young and wrinkle free.

Yet, ageing is a natural, slow and irreversible process of evolution which cannot be stopped. Nevertheless, women – and increasingly men – are flocking to beauticians, chemists and clinics in search of quick fix cures in order to turn back the clock. Pharmacists and plastic surgeons have become the new gurus to whom people entrust their most exposed and most fragile organ - the skin on their face.

The conventional approach to anti ageing has always been a symptomatic one, focusing solely on the visible symptoms like wrinkles, sagging features etc. However, even a surgical face lift provides a temporary solution only (apart from possible serious side effects) requiring later follow ups or even corrective measures.

Natural Medicine has no cure for ageing either. However, it is able to offer a gentle long term approach to tired skin, fine lines and even deep wrinkles. As it takes into account our general constitution as well as the present state of health, it offers us the chance to become actively involved in managing our health and subtly but profoundly changing the way we look.

The techniques explained in this manual will provide you with an easy to learn tool that can be learned in minutes and applied immediately.

Have fun and success in taking care of yourself in an effective and easy – yet rewarding – way!

Skin deep

Our skin is not only our largest organ, it also weighs twice as much as our brain. It completely wraps around our body - supple enough to allow movement but, at the same time tough enough to shield us against injury.

It protects the internal organs and retains essential fluids while resisting infection and damaging radiation by the sunlight.
It keeps our internal temperatures constant by conserving heat or cooling the body when necessary.

If that's not enough, our skin takes care of the excretion of toxins and waste material that cannot pass through the kidneys and distributes nutrients and oxygen to the nerves and glands, hair and nails.

Last, but not least, it allows any sensory information to travel to the brain – be it pleasant or unpleasant like pain.

To do all this, the skin is fitted with unique

qualities – hair follicles to get sebum to the surface, nerve receptors that are acutely sensitive and elastic tissues capable of expanding by 50 per cent. In addition, it is extremely adaptable to climates and temperatures, to our moods and our age.

Taking into consideration that our skin is the most expressive and most exposed part of our body, it is only understandable that women – and increasingly men – are concerned with keeping their skin healthy and glowing while - at the same time - trying to delay the onset of wrinkles as much as possible.

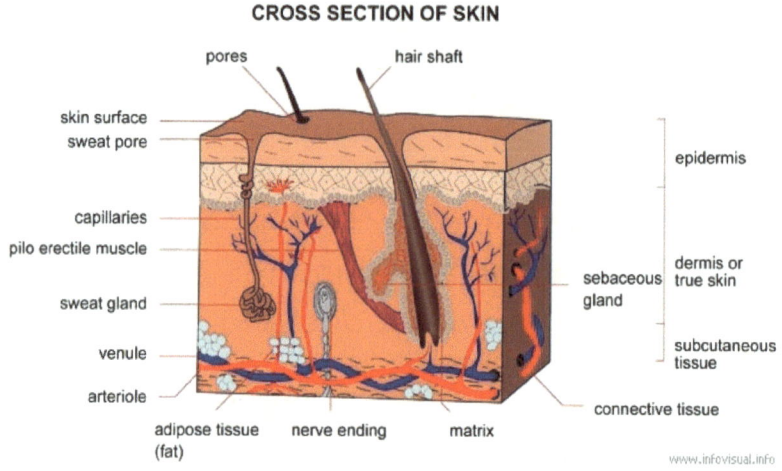

CROSS SECTION OF SKIN

The foundation of the skin is the hypodermis containing fat cells, blood vessels and nerve fibres. Above that, we find the skin's support system, the dermis. It not only holds blood vessels, nerve ends, hair follicles, sebaceous and sweat glands and connective tissue but - most importantly - it contains collagen, a protein that gives the skin its bounce and vitality by providing structure and support.

The fact that collagen production declines with age usually results in tired, sagging skin and eventually wrinkles. While in a teenager's skin the cells are regenerating at a record speed of around 28 days, this will slow down to about 45 days for a woman in her fifties. Furthermore, menopause might bring a sharp decline in estrogen production leading to a fall of sebum. Consequently, water evaporates easier, resulting in drier skin. The top layer – the epidermis – becomes about 20 per cent thinner than during teenage years; the distribution of fatty cells becomes uneven, drooping jowls and a heavier chin might be appearing.

Western Medicine and Traditional Chinese Medicine

In order to understand the effect of 'Facial Acupressure' on the face and the body as well, it is important to appreciate the difference between Western Medicine and TCM.

The conventional Western view of the body emphasizes the physical structures and components that interact in a very subtle and complex manner. Anatomy and physiology map these structures from the largest – bones, muscles, skin and so on – to the smallest – the cells and their components. This structural map forms the basis of the model of cause and effect that dominates Western Medicine.

Traditional Chinese Medicine (TCM) engages a very different model. It considers components of process rather than of structure. The human body is seen first and foremost as an Energy system in which various substances interact to create the whole physical organism.

For the appreciation of the effect of acupressure and acupuncture on our body, two fundamental concepts of TCM must be explained.

Yin and Yang

There is a variety of interpretations of this concept – the most simple one being the comparison with a mountain under the midday sun. As one side is in bright sunlight (Yang), the other side enjoys cooling shade (Yin). As such, Yin characteristics are said to be cool, dark, receptive, quiet, preserving and solid, Yang is said to relate more to warm, light, extroverted, active and moving aspects.

It is most important to understand that Yin and Yang might be opposites - but only in relation to each other. One cannot be defined without the other, they are two aspects of the same phenomenon and form a description, not a judgment.

Every second of our life we are surrounded by the manifestation of Yin and Yang – as night (Yin) recedes, the sun (Yang) rises and warms the earth; reaching its peak during midday it gradually fades during late afternoon into the night (Yin) again. In the same way, (human) life changes from youth

(Yang) to older age until it returns to the earth (Yin) from which new life will be formed.

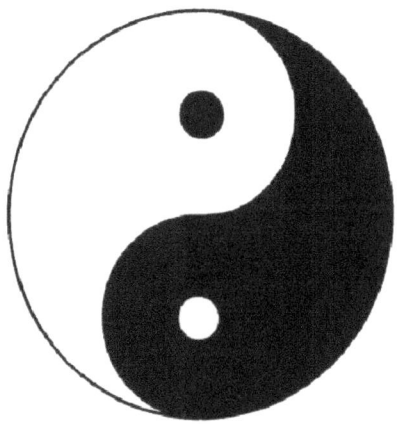

TCM states that as long as there is balance, health will prevail; any kind of dis-ease is the result of an imbalance between Yin and Yang. When one becomes domineering it will weaken the other.

For example, an increase in body heat (Yang) will dry out our body fluids (Yin) whose main task is to cool the body – subsequently, the body might get overly hot, resulting in a flushed face, dry mouth, cracked lips and perhaps developing later into headache, sore throat, constipation, restlessness and insomnia.

In order to restore balance between Yin and Yang, acupressure or acupuncture is applied to specific points and areas on the body and face; these points exert influence on our Life Force, called 'Ch'i' in TCM context.

What is Ch'i?

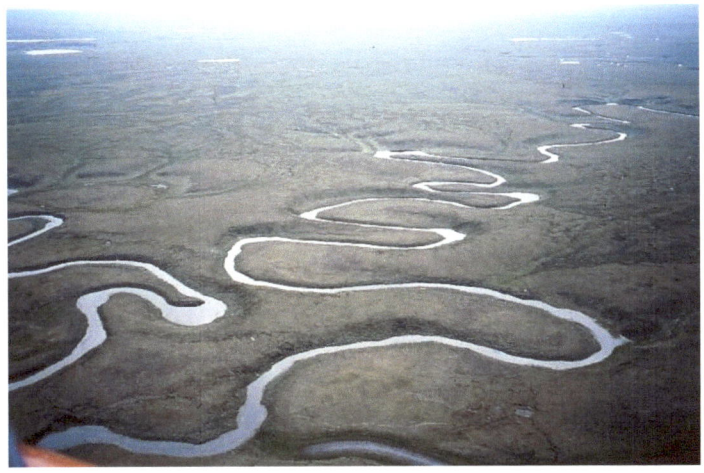

TCM is primarily based on the notion that every living being – humans, animals, plants, in fact the whole Universe – is animated by a certain Life Force, the Ch'i. It is the life behind the atom – the Energy found in all forms of matter and is concentrated in living organisms. In order to nourish our tissues and organs and keep them well functioning it should flow through our body not too fast and not too slow – similar to a river meandering through meadows and mountains.

If Ch'i is blocked or stagnates, the Yin/Yang balance is disturbed and our cells are not supported. This might result in physical. mental or emotional illness. For example, it might manifest in headache, chronic fatigue and dizziness, lack of concentration or nervousness.

The first area to detect disturbed or unbalanced Ch'i is our emotional system – are we feeling tense, restless, irritable, constantly tired or even angry? By detecting the pattern behind the symptoms we are able to correct the flow of the Ch'i in order to re-establish balance – before the imbalance manifests itself in pain or disease.

How do we correct our Ch'i?

Our Life Force runs through a complex network of channels (Meridians) that link with each other building an endless circuit of Energy; at the same time connecting the interior with the exterior, the organs with the tissues and so on.

This Meridian system consists of 12 main channels running mainly along the long axis of the body, and 8 extraordinary Meridians. Each of the 12 main channels pertains to a specific organ and influences the Energy of that organ significantly; however, via collaterals and small branches other parts of the body are influenced as well.

The function of the Meridians is to provide even circulation of the Ch'i throughout the body, thus nourishing the tissues and linking up the whole body in order to keep the internal organs, the skin (our largest external organ), the limbs, muscles, tendons and bones intact and function as one organic integrity.

For the purpose of correcting the flow of the Ch'i, we are able to access the Energy via specific points along the Meridians – points where we can tap the Ch'i. Whether we use needles (Acupuncture) or finger pressure (Acupressure) or heat (Moxibustion), any kind of impact on one or several Acupuncture points will cause subtle changes within the Energy system with consequent physical and emotional effects.

What is 'Facial Acupressure'?

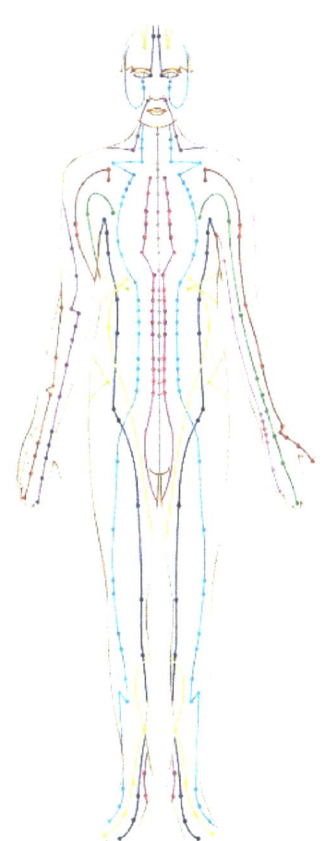

Almost all Meridians begin or end in the face – the Stomach Meridian starts below the eye, the Gall Bladder Meridian starts at the outer canthus of the eye, the Urinary Bladder Meridian starts at the inner eye, the Large Intestine Meridian ends at the nostrils, the Small Intestine Meridian ends at the temples, the Ren Meridian ends in the cleft on the chin, the Du Meridian ends on the philtrum close to the upper lip and so on. As all starting and ending points of Meridians are perceived as having an especially strong effect on the body's Energy it is only logical that any manipulation of these points will result in a noticeable change within our Energy system.

This change is manifested in two ways:
Acupressure on the particular points in the prescribed way will create warmth which converts into a minute electrical charge. This charge feeds the muscles, nerves and lymphatic system while clearing any blockages.

Some acupuncture points regulate the endocrine response to perform homoeostasis in the body resulting in the production of hormones and reinforcement of new cells - consequently, blood and Energy circulation within the face are increased, lines will soften, tissue becomes tighter and the face returns to a healthy glow.

At the same time, not only the facial Energy is being stimulated but all the respective Meridians as well which results in an overall shift in well being. When internal Energy is flowing easily and undisturbed, the body's systems operate harmoniously with one another – which naturally results in improved health.

The Face as a Mirror of the Organs

In TCM diagnosis, the face is closely examined in order to detect any imbalance between the different organ systems.

If the Energy of the Kidney is insufficient this will show in a greyish complexion, dark circles under the eyes, puffy eyelids and perhaps a bony appearance – physical/emotional symptoms may include lumbago, frequent urination, weak lower limbs, a dry throat and a tendency towards being too fearful.

A deficiency of Ch'i in the Lung will result in a pale, almost translucent complexion and probably rather dry skin with an early appearance of small wrinkles – physically/emotionally, this imbalance could result in a tendency towards frequent colds or cough, sore throat, pain along the outer side of the arm and a lingering feeling of sadness

A disturbance in the Liver Energy might be apparent in a greenish complexion, tense facial muscles, yellowish eyes and pigmentation – physical/emotional symptoms could be headache/migraine, painful joints and tendons, a feeling of congestion in the chest and being prone to getting easily angered and frustrated.

If there is a deficiency in the Spleen Energy, the face will have a waxy appearance, heavy eye bags, sagging facial muscles and dark areas around the lips – physically/emotionally, it could manifest in belching, abdominal distension, menstrual issues, edema, loose stools, a general sluggishness and a tendency to becoming constantly worried.

An imbalance in the Heart Energy is expressed in a red face, but pale lips, wrinkled skin and shrunken facial muscles – pain in the cardiac region, insomnia, night sweat and loss of concentration and a tendency towards getting easily overexcited might be the physical/emotional symptoms.

Positive Effects
of Facial Acupressure

- Improves muscle tone and tightens the skin

- Eliminates or reduces puffiness and 'eye bags'

- Eliminates or reduces double chin

- Moisturizes skin by increasing circulation of blood and lymph to the face

- Eliminates fine lines – reduces deeper wrinkles

- Slows the ageing process from within

- Increases collagen production

- Reduces or smoothes acne scars

- Improves facial color by increasing peripheral circulation

- Relaxes the entire face, body and mind

- Promotes overall health and well being

Acupressure versus Surgical Facelift

The following thoughts refer to surgical facelifts for 'cosmetic' reasons only – there is no doubt that a surgical intervention for a disfigured face or features that influence the respective person psychologically are a blessing and not the subject of this considerations.

For almost everyone, a **surgical facelift** is expected to eliminate lines, firm sagging tissue but also to restore beauty and youth to the face.

It is important to understand that plastic surgery cannot stop the ageing process nor can it prevent the clock from ticking. A successful operation might result in a more rested look - however, it can also change the character of the person, giving an artificial image.

With surgery, some lines might be eliminated but it will not restore life and vitality of the skin. Furthermore, it usually is not a one shot procedure but requires a repetition within eighteen months to five years after the initial surgery.

Like any operation, a conventional facelift carries a risk of complication. No matter how skilled the physician, surgery (anesthesia etc.) interrupts the Energy System of the whole body – it is not an isolated procedure limited to the face.

Added to the above are the cost of hospitalization, bandages, discoloration and time for recovering etc.

The Acupressure Facelift does not involve big expenses, hospitals, pain and risks; it only requires determination and discipline and a bit of time. It is totally natural, something everybody can do him/herself and for others, at any chosen time, independently.

Dry and lackluster skin and lines are not just the signs of getting older. They also represent stress and neglect, lack of sleep or exercise and poor diet. To attempt to deal with these signs exclusively through surgical removal means essentially denying the body the chance to confront any problem in a natural way – one is dealing with the effect but ignoring the cause.

Acupressure treats the underlying cause of why someone is aging, instead of masking the outward symptoms and allowing further decline and dysfunction to continue within the body.

While a surgical facelift is only able to tighten the skin, acupressure/acupuncture increases blood circulation to the face, promotes collagen production and enhances muscle tone and elasticity.

Face Lines

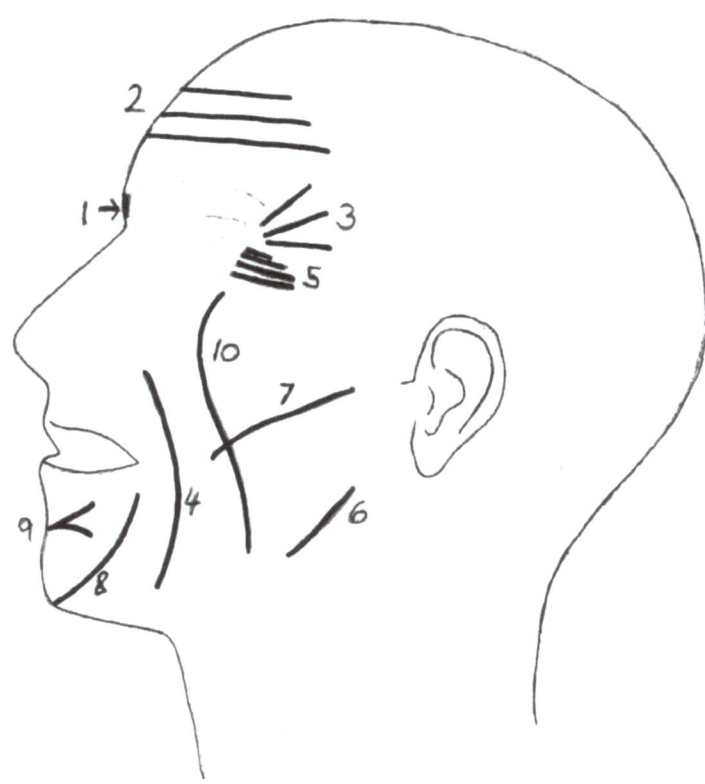

1 – Frowning Lines	**6 – Moon Line**
2 – Thinking Lines	**7 – Mars line**
3 – Venus Lines	**8 – Social Line**
4 – Provocation Lines	**9 – Jupiter Line**
5 – Weather Element Lines	**10- Mercury Line**

Most of the facial lines are caused by weak muscles, overuse or natural ageing.

Reduced metabolism and circulation hinder the sufficient nutrition of the skin. The fat deposits which keep the skin tight and the reduced function of the sebaceous glands with age cause the tissue to sag or become dry and therefore lined.

Face Muscles

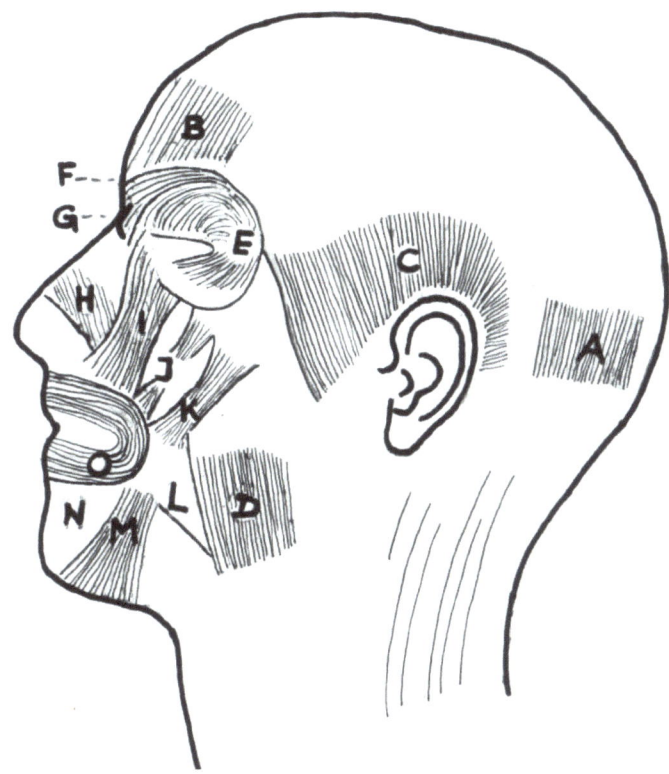

A - Occipital Muscle

B - Frontal Occipital Muscle (Frowning Lines)

C - Ear Muscle (tightening of eye wrinkles (Venus Lines)

   and cheek (Mars Line)

D - Masseter Muscle (double chin, tightening of cheek)

E - Orbicularis Oculi (eye bags, eye wrinkles)

F - Oculi Corrigating Muscle (tightening of eyelid)

G - Procerus Muscles (nasal lines correction)

H - Nasal/ Lever Muscle (firming the nose triangle)

I - Upper Lip Muscle (lifting corners of mouth)

J - Zygomaticus Muscle (firming cheek and lifting corners of mouth)

K - Zygomaticus Majorale (same as J)

L - Risorius Muscle ('laughing muscle', tightens neck)

M - Depressor Anguli oris (double chin)

N.- Under Lip Muscle (tightens chin)

O.- Orbicularis Oris (lifting corners of mouth)

Each of the muscles can be stimulated separately – either by acupuncture (placing the needle into the centre of the muscle) or by acupressure (massaging the respective points).

Tips for Massaging

The points for acupressure are the same as for acupuncture; however acupressure does not involve needles but applies finger force on the respective points or areas in order to clear any obstruction within the Meridians. Consequently, any stagnation is forced to escape and circulation can set in again.

How?

Before starting any massage on your face (or somebody else's face) wash your hands and face, followed by the application of a light moisturizing cream.

Sit or stand in front of a mirror in order to control the correct location of the points.

Do not pull the skin or push too hard; just apply **firm pressure first** (either with your Index or middle finger) on the point followed by **very small** circles until you feel some tingling or slight soreness.

Hold the pressure for ca, 10 seconds, then release for 10 seconds – repeat about 5 times followed by lightly tapping the area with your finger tips

When changing to another point don't drag over the skin, instead release the pressure before repositioning your hand and continue to exert gentle but firm pressure on the respective points.

Most of the points are bilateral – located on both the right and left side of the face. Unless otherwise indicated massage both sides simultaneously with each hand.
As the Meridian system has a directional flow; try to follow the indicated direction of massage - however, if in doubt, massage in both directions (even method).

While massaging try to be relaxed and calm; breathe deeply and rhythmically; do not pull up your shoulders. If they are tight roll them up and down, backward and forward in order to reduce tension. Never be in a hurry.

When?

It does not matter so much when it is done – as long it is done at all!

However, within the Chinese system, the morning time (before noon) is favoured as the body produces most hormones at this time of the day.

Equally, it can be done in the evening to unwind after a long day – combining it with the usual facial routine.

How often

In order to achieve best results one should do the routine at least once every day, for one month. After that it is sufficient to gear down to two to three times a week in order to maintain the achieved result.

How long

The whole procedure might take up approximately 15 to 20 minutes – each point should be stimulated for about a minute.

Questions and Answers

Will it be for ever?

The benefits of Facial Acupressure are permanent as long as the massage is maintained. After about thirty days of daily massage the muscles and skin of the face will improve to the point that three sessions a week are sufficient for maintenance purpose. Facial muscles respond to exercise in the same way as muscles of the rest of the body.

If stopped, will the face suddenly age?

If the massage is stopped for a few weeks (after having done it for at least thirty days) nothing much will happen. However, if nothing is done for a long period of time the face might return to its previous look.

Is it possible to concentrate on special areas only?

For specific areas, some extra time might be beneficial. However, for maximum overall results, the entire massage should be completed first.

Can it help seventy-year-old skin that is already wrinkled?

It will definitely make a difference. Facial muscles are muscles, no matter what age. However, as in all complementary medicine modalities, it is known that the longer a condition exists, the longer it takes to restore it normalcy. One would have to be a bit more patient but the result is well worth it.

Any conditions under which not to do the massage?

Any blemishes, injuries or cuts should better be left alone; also, after surgery, nothing should disturb the healing process before the respective area is completely healed.

Will the massage eliminate acne scars?

Unfortunately, scarring is a 'permanent' condition. However, by invigorating the circulation and revitalizing the muscles, the skin becomes healthier, takes on a natural color and fills out. These changes tend to make the scars less visible.

Does the Facial Acupressure work for men too?

In this respect, there is no difference between male and female facial skin and muscles – the result will be an improved muscle tone, minimizing or even eliminating wrinkles and a healthy glow.

Can it be done even before developing wrinkles?

TCM places great importance on prevention of disease – that attitude is the same for facial acupressure: by regularly massaging the face, circulation is kept strong, channels stay clear of obstruction and blockages and muscles will remain supple. Consequently, the appearance of wrinkles is delayed and the face will look much younger.

Does the massage eliminate aging spots or sun spots?

Basically no, but it may render them much less visible as circulation to the skin is being restored. Often, stressed and over worked people start to change their life style after starting the facial massage – they change their eating habits, do more exercise and overall take better care of themselves. As a result, they look and feel better, the previously tired and pale skin radiates so the age spots become much less visible.

What causes 'under eye bags' and can they be treated as well?

The muscles below the eyes weaken and break down allowing fat particles to herniated through them and push outward. By massaging these areas the muscles around the eyes regain tone and firmness and are therefore more effective in holding back the fat.

The following pages
show a detailled description
of all points for
'Facelift by Acupressure'.

Point 1

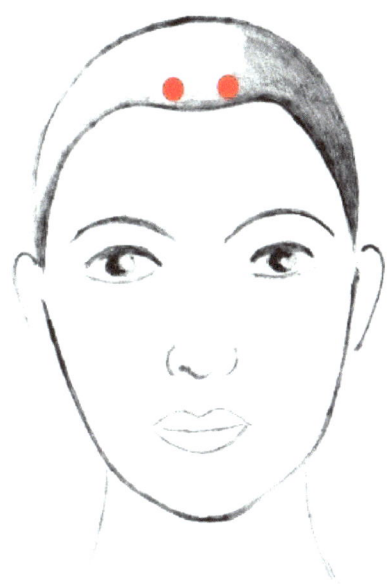

Ub 3 – Mei Chong

Located about 1 cm within the hairline – directly above the medial end of the eyebrows.

This starting point of the program opens the flow of Energy down into your face. The thin muscles in this area of the scalp and forehead will be relaxed and invigorated by the massage.

Use firm pressure and make very small **inward** circles.

In TCM, this point is also used to treat simple headaches and relaxes the eyes.

Point 2

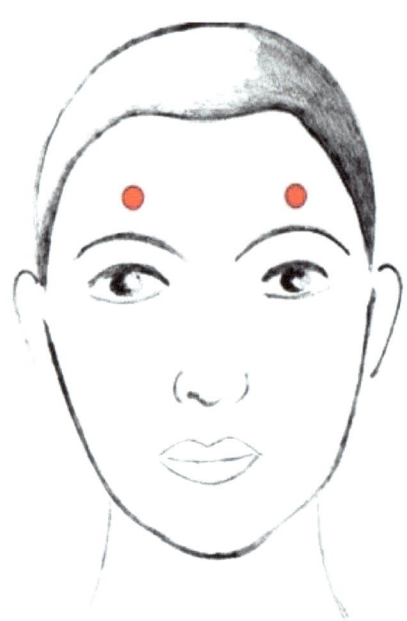

Gb 14 – YangBai

Located directly above the centre of each eye when looking straight, about 2 cm above the eyebrows.

This point is very relaxing, working on the skin and muscles of the forehead. The muscles in that area support the layers of the skin that have a tendency to form deep lines. Stimulation of this point will be building up the muscle tissue.

Use firm pressure and make very small **inward** circles.

In TCM, this point is often used for eye problems, frontal headache and insomnia.

Point 3

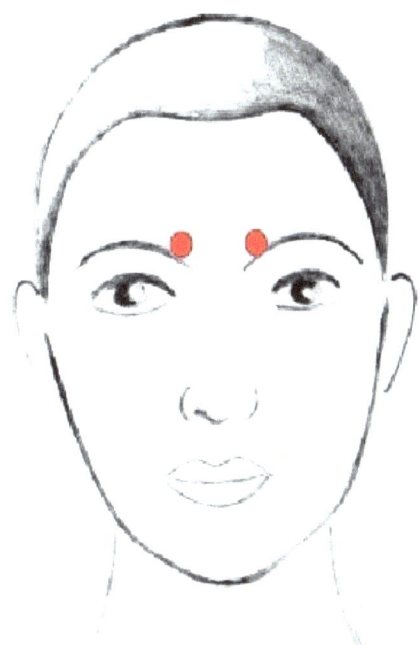

Ub 2 – ZanZhu

Located at the medial end of the eyebrows.

Activating this point stimulates the flow of Energy around the eyes, along the nose and into the centre of the face.

Make small **inward** circles, being careful not to push against the eyes.

In TCM, this point is traditionally used for discomfort around the eyes, headache and has an effect on the sinuses.

Point 4

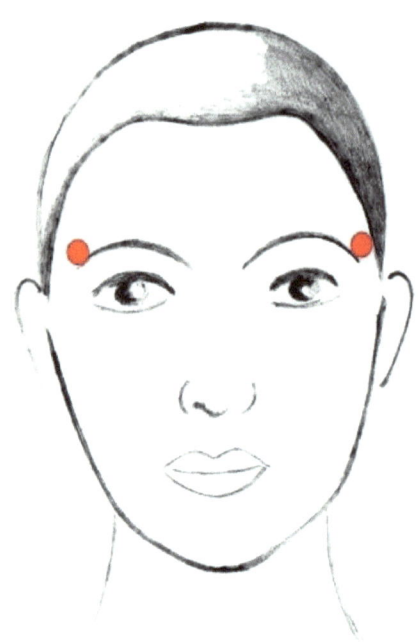

Sj 23 – Sizhu Kong

Located in the depression at the lateral end of the eyebrows

This point works on the delicate muscle structure above the eyes and temples; it is especially beneficial for 'crow's feet' because it helps to fill out the tissue under which the creases tend to develop.

Make small **outward** circles. Remember to stay relaxed and do not pull up your shoulders; if you do – stop, roll your shoulders backward and forward and start again.

In TCM, this point is used as well for sudden headache, dizziness and dry eyes.

Point 5

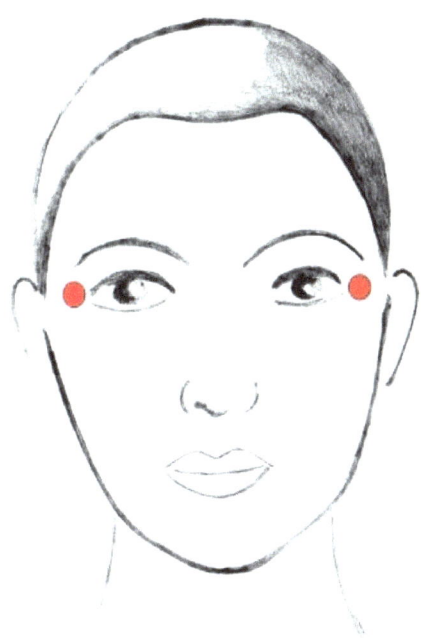

Wai Ming (Extra point)

Located at the outside corner of the eyes; this is where 'crow's feet' start to emerge

Massaging this point enhances circulation and Energy to the eyes and the area of the eye sockets; consequently, the muscles are toned and the skin becomes supple.

Make small **outward** circles; be careful not to push against the eye. Feel for the little depression in the muscle and use firm pressure.

In TCM, this Extra point is also used for irritated or dry eyes.

Point 6

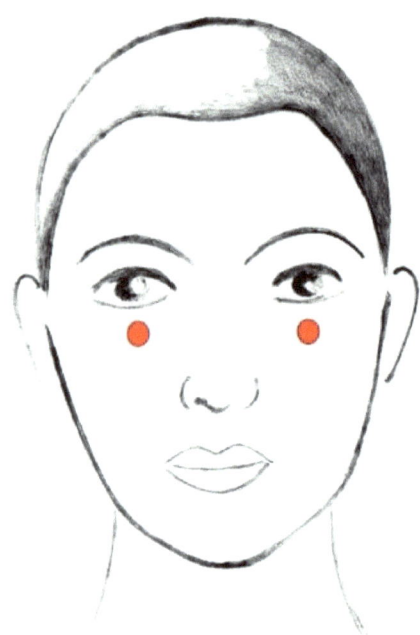

St 1 – Cheng Qi

Massaging this point helps to restore the muscle tissue to prevent 'eye bags' from developing.

Make small **outward** circles; do not press on the eyes.

In TCM, this point treats conjunctivitis and any kind of eye strain.

Point 7

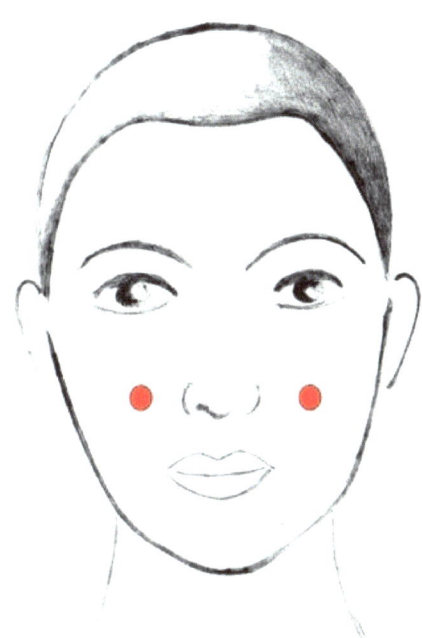

St 3 – Juliao

Located further down directly below the previous point, in an even line with the nostrils.

This point works on the large cheek muscle, filling out sunken tissue and restoring the natural angles of your face. Circulation is especially enhanced as well resulting in a healthy glow.

Make small **outward** circles.

In TCM, this point has a beneficial effect on the sinuses and on any vision issues.

Point 8

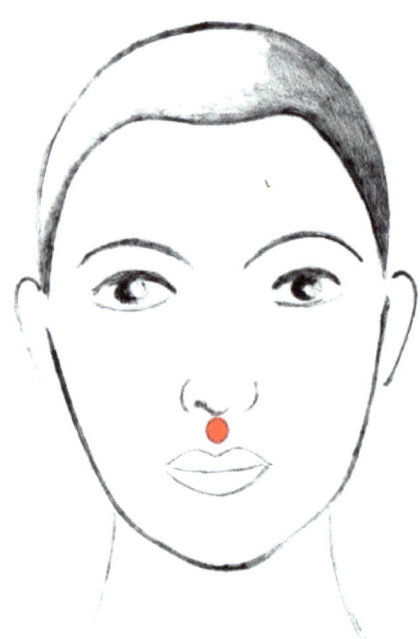

Ren Zhong (Extra point)

Located below the nose, in the upper third of the philtrum

Stimulating this area is helpful for the vertical lines that appear below the nose above the upper lip.

Make small **clockwise** circles with firm pressure

In TCM, this is known as the 'Emergency Point' as it is often used for fainting, dizziness and nausea.

At this point,
it might be advisable

to take a break:

shake out the hands,

let them fall on your lap,

roll your shoulders forward

and backward

and take a few deep breaths

Point 9

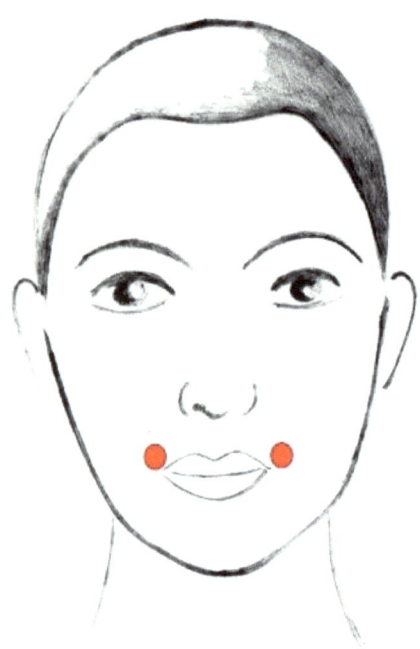

St 4 – Dicang

Located above your upper lip about 1 cm from the outside corners of the mouth.

This point as well influences the small wrinkles around the corners of the mouth.

Make small **outward** circles with firm pressure.

In TCM, this point is used in the connection with facial paralysis.

Point 10

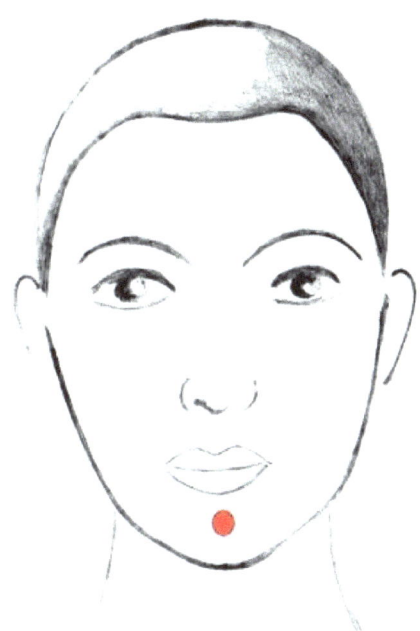

Ren 24 – Cheng Jiang

Located midway between the lower lip and the chin.

Massaging this point helps to lessen the small wrinkles that might develop on the chin. It is a gateway point that channels circulation and Energy up to the area of the mouth and face.

Make small **clockwise** circles.

In TCM, it is also used for facial paralysis and toothache.

Point 11

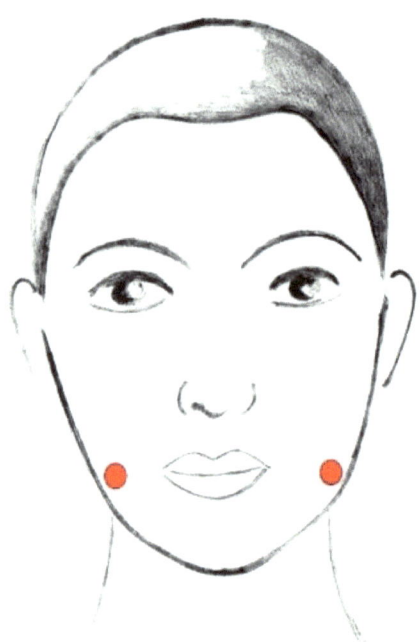

St 6 – Jiache

Located on the big muscle at the hinge of the jaw (open your mouth slightly)

This point is especially useful for tension in the jaw and enhances the entire Energy flow into the face. It can and should be massaged whenever one feels tense or stressed during the day.

Make small circles **toward the back of the head.**

In TCM, this point is well known for its effect on tooth ache or jaw pain.

Point 12

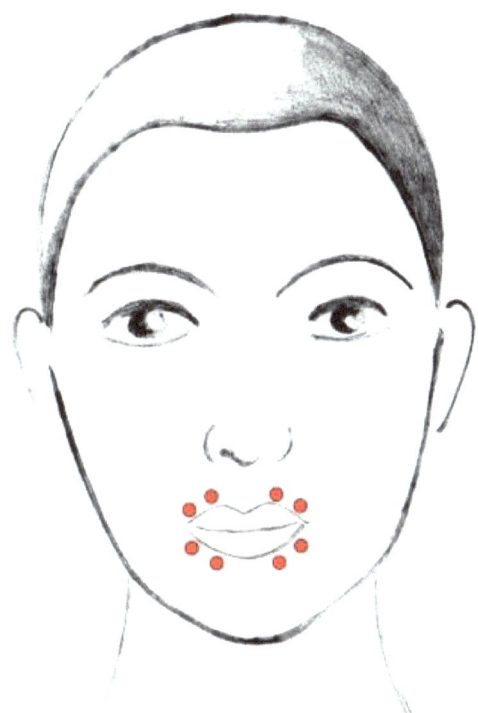

These points do not carry names in TCM

They are located above the upper lip and below the lower lip, about 1 cm from the corner of the mouth away.

They are especially effective for the small lines above and below the lips.

Make small **outward** circles.

Chin Slap

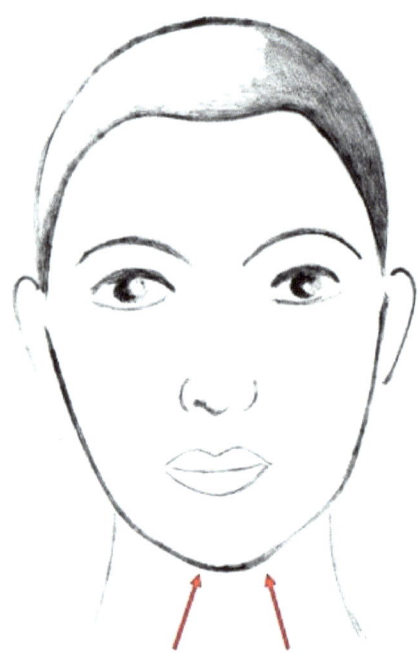

Do some rhythmic slapping on the chin and tissue that often tends to sag just below your chin.

Stick your chin out and use the backs of both hands alternatively to do a stimulating massage.

There is no need to slap hard – just firmly enough to feel the circulation being stimulated. Do this for about 30 seconds.

Point 13

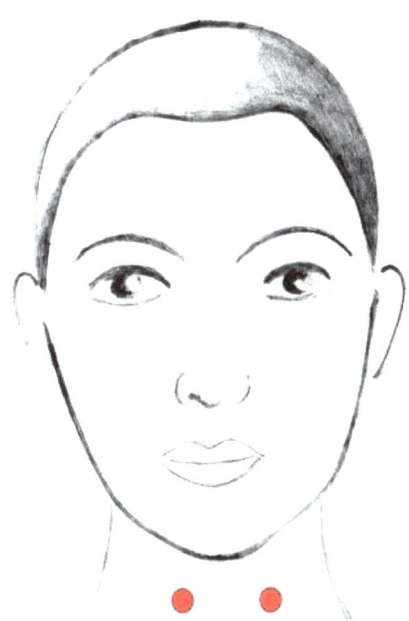

St 9 – Ren Ying

Bring your fingers to your throat midway on your neck at both side of the wind pipe. It's easier to find when leaning back the head a little.

This point stimulates the area of the thyroid glands and generates Energy throughout the whole body. It helps to firm and tone the muscles and tissues around the throat

Please, only press and circle **lightly** for about 20 to 30 seconds.

In TCM, this point influences swallowing, speech and breathing issues.

Point 14

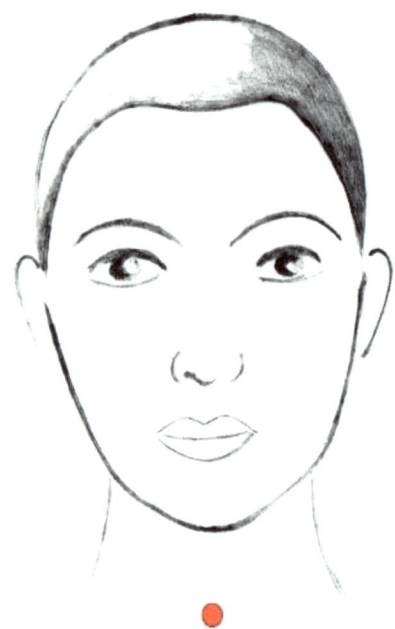

Ren 22 – Tian Tu

Located in the notch of the bone at the base of the throat

This point opens up important pathways of Energy into the neck, head and body.

Stay on the bone and make **small** circles; be careful not to push into your wind pipe.

In TCM, this is a very effective point for sudden hoarseness, cough and phlegm in the throat.

Points Summary

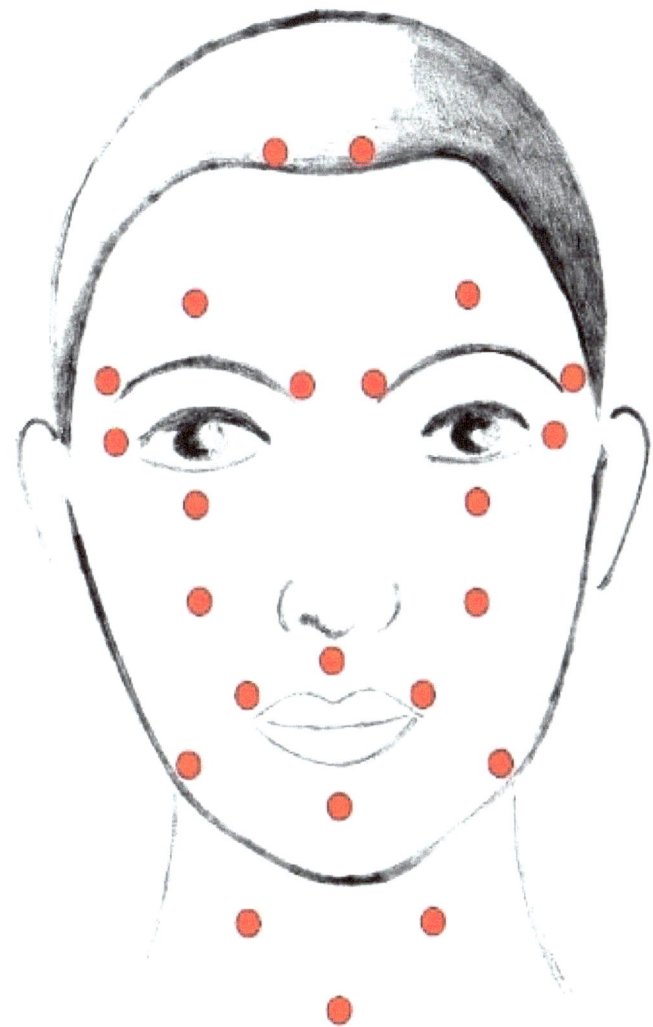

Special Cosmetic Points

The following two points on the Large Intestine (Li) Meridian are not located on the face but on the body. They are key points for stimulating the Energy in the face and influence the digestion as well.

Point 15 - Li 4 – Hegu

Located on each hand in the soft 'webbed' tissue where thumb and forefinger come together. Gripping one hand with thumb and forefinger of the other hand a tender point is felt – use deep **circular** massage for about a minute. Then alternate hands.

This point is one of the main points to stimulate Energy in the whole body.

In TCM, it is especially effective for sore throat, fever and any abdominal distension.

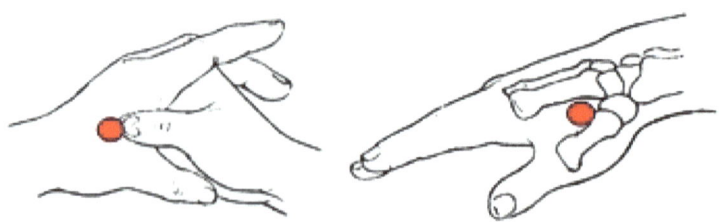

Point 16 - Li 11 – Chize

Located on the elbow at the base of the elbow crease – the arm has to be flexed.

Use your thumb to push into the soft area until you feel a slight tingling; then massage in a **circular** motion for about a minute.

This point is one of the main points to influence the quality of the skin.

In TCM, it is primarily used for digestive disorders, high blood pressure and allergies.

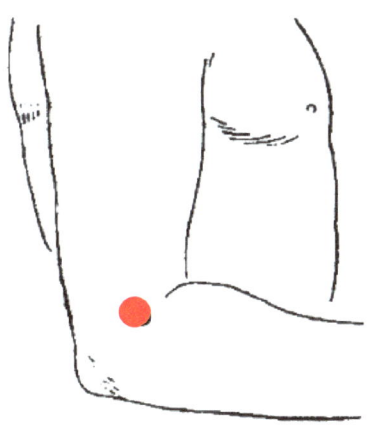

Other Influences

The Facelift by Acupressure is a simple and relaxing method that can be easily integrated into a busy schedule. It will not only improve skin tone and diminish lines and wrinkles but will be beneficial for the whole body, the complete Energy system. As a natural consequence, one becomes more health conscious in a holistic way.

However, beauty basically reflects also the inner well being – therefore sleep, relaxation, wholesome nutrition and a positive attitude are of great influence. No beauty regimen will erase the signs of an abusive life style.

Sleep

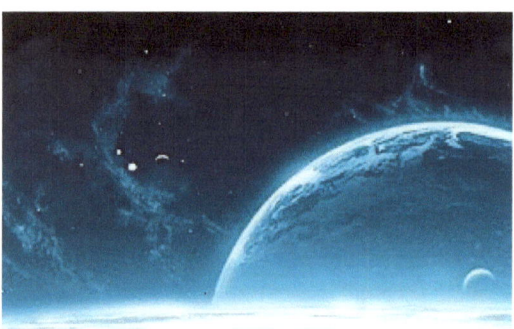 There are no fast and fixed rules for the individual amount of sleep; however, lack of sleep or an irregular sleep pattern over a prolonged

period of time will show first and foremost in the face.

As babies, we could drop off to sleep at any time during the day and for almost any length of time – however our lifestyle is now characterized by a 24hour society which leaves most of us sleep deprived; dark circles, saggy eyelids and a drained and tired looking skin are the price.

Insomnia has become the number one complaint – not falling asleep or waking up at odd times during the night, snoring or not being able to switch off the mind – sleep disorders have even led to the establishment of specialized sleep clinics.

Considering that sleep is vital for the regeneration of damaged and tired cells, the importance of enough and regular rest in order to keep the skin healthy is easy to understand.

Stress

Our face shows everything – whether a child is struggling with a difficult math calculation or we are stuck in the traffic before an important meeting, the emotional or physiological distress will leave its marks in creases, wrinkles and furrows somewhere on our face and neck.

Everyone's face responds in a similar way. However, while teenager's skin will bounce back after the stress has subsided, adult skin has become short of springy tissue – therefore hanging on to the stress, embedding it in the dermis. Coupled with the general slower regeneration of cells and the long term effects of our life style it is easy to see why stress might add years to our body and skin.

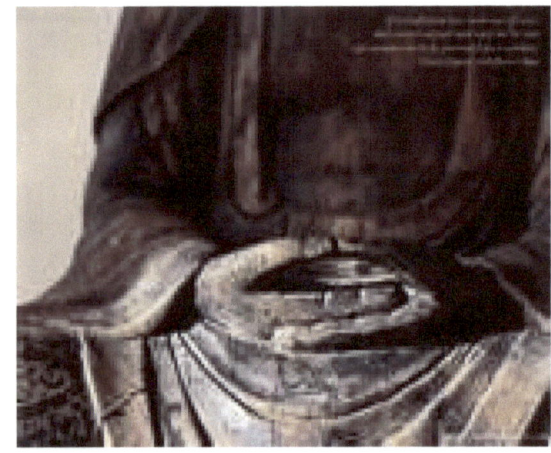

Relaxation – in whatever form – should be a part of

the daily routine. Some of the most effective ways of conscious relaxation go back thousands of years. Yoga, meditation or visualization are the three most popular and effective methods which can be practiced by themselves or incorporated in an individual daily relaxation program.

Whether it is deep breathing or meditating or listening to your favorite music, there should be at least 45 minutes daily reserved just for that.

Posture and Attitude

If we constantly think of gravity pulling everything down – exactly this will be the result. Whatever we think and feel will eventually come into existence. Why not think of gravity as an orderly power in space and time which assists us by lending support and structure and keeps us upright.

It depends on us how we wish to place ourselves between 'Heaven and Earth' – bent over with hanging shoulders, and drawn

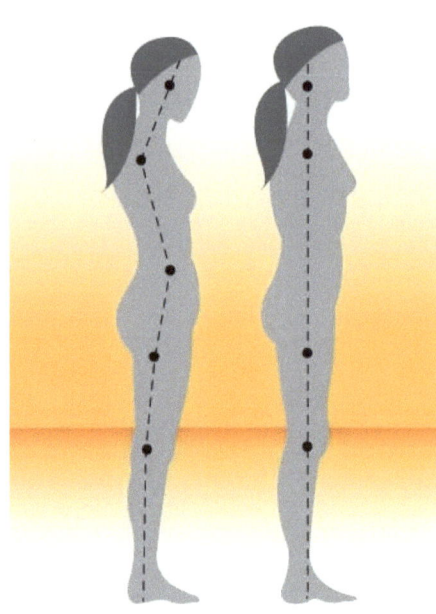

facial features or upright with a straight spine and a head held high Leave your neck relaxed and resist the urge to scrunch up your shoulders. A better and stronger posture will not only effect your physical appearance but also your emotional constitution as well as minor aches and pains.

It really pays to constantly observe the way how we walk, stand and especially sit; since a great deal of time is spent in front of computers, the occurrence of migraine and tension headache has increased tremendously.

Nutrition

There are thousands of books about diet and 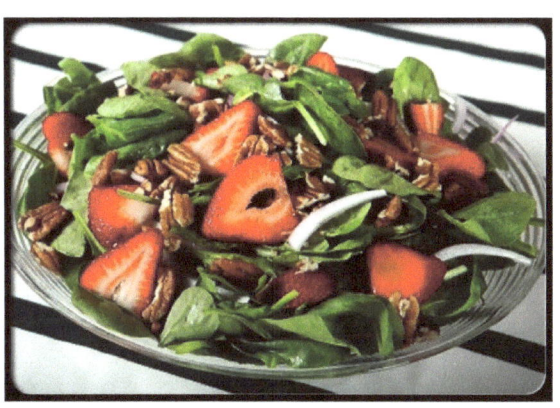 food and some are even contradicting each other; therefore it is only by individual experience of the effects on the face and body which enables one to decide for a certain diet.

Whether being vegetarian, meat eater or raw food lover, there are some undesirable ingredients that apply to any kind of nutrition – too much sugar and wheat (affects the tissue), too much salt (may lead to swollen eyes), chemicals and additives (cause bloating and allergies, prevent weight loss etc.) and too little water.

While **dehydration** in other organs of the body can cause a whole spectrum of issues that are mostly invisible, the effect of dehydrated skin manifests itself in obvious wrinkles and bulges.

As our body consists two thirds of water, insufficient hydration prevents it from effectively eliminating toxins through the kidney and colon – therefore the skin has to work especially hard to release them through the pores.

Subsequently, the skin looses elasticity, becomes dry and is more prone to infections. The elasticity and suppleness of the skin has to come from within.

No amount of moisturizer will compensate for not drinking enough (six to eight glasses) water.

Emotions

Last, but not least: Everyone knows that a negative attitude to life is mirrored in the facial expression.

Constant worries or doubts, repressed anger, bitterness and a fearful outlook will lead to tensed muscles in the jaw, narrow lips, sagging tissue and frowning lines which, over a period of time, 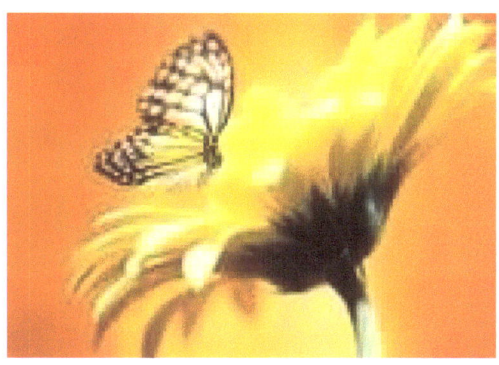 will change the physiognomy tremendously.

No amount of creams or chemical procedures is able to erase the ensuing effect.

The best guarantee for a youthful face might just be a happy constitution, a curious mind and a forgiving heart, not being attached to past hurt but looking forward to the joys of the future.

It is the healthy balance between accepting and adjusting to what can't be changed and actively influencing where change is possible that will facilitate an inner equilibrium which will ultimately be the best foundation for a youthful looking face – no matter what age.

About the Author

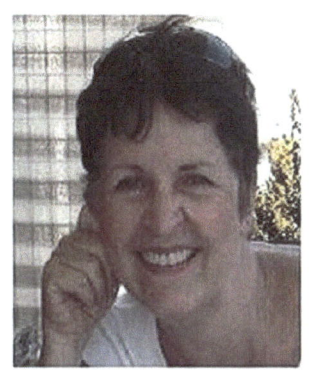

Apart from an early interest in the Art and Culture of Asia (and the Cuisine...), nothing had prepared me for the life that today fills my heart with so much joy and gratitude.

My professional background was in languages but most of all, in Design (Graphic, Fashion, Furniture, Interior) and painting. By now, we have been living more than 34 years in SE Asia; those very challenging first years in a foreign – albeit fascinating – part of the world had a truly profound effect on our life, molding me to a great extent into the person I am today.

After 7 years living in Asia I got interested in Acupressure which was followed by many years of professional studies of Acupuncture, Reiki, BACH Flowers, JinShinJyutsu, EFT, Personality Analysis etc. It was a definite career change – which deeply influenced our family life as well. Throughout these years, the theory of the Five Elements has influenced me the most.

The wisdom within this philosophy enables me to discover ever new layers within a person – be it physical or emotional, be it in a child or an adult, whether it concerns health or behavior.

Most important, it allows me to view every person with respect – neither good nor bad – and to know that we are all perfect - at any given time.

My work with my clients and patients is based on a gentle guidance through the demands of life incorporating counseling as well as the Healing Modality that is most suitable for the respective person, the issue in question, at that particular time; it is important to me that one is always aware of his/her self responsibility. Naturally, I consult and cooperate with representatives of Conventional Medicine whenever this is required or desired and give advice on nutritional issues as well.

A great deal of my time and effort is spent in constant further education of all Healing Modalities. I live and work in Singapore

Qualifications

Traditional Chinese Medicine - Dipl. Ac.

JinShinJyutsu - Practitioner graduated

BACH Flowers - Practioner certified

EFT (Emotional Freedom Technique) - certified

Reiki - Master and Teacher (Usui)

Karuna Reiki - Master and Teacher

Feng Shui

Personality Analysis

I Ching - all graduated under
GrandMaster Raymond Lo

Publications

Facelift by Acupressure
on www.Amazon.com

The Yin and Yang of Food and Nutrition
on www.Amazon.com

Life in Balance

Alternative Ways to Holistic Healing

for Body, Mind and Spirit

www.lifebalance.com.sg

www.ingramcontent.com/pod-product-compliance
Lightning Source LLC
Chambersburg PA
CBHW050809290526
45792CB00001B/48